GLP Blueprint
Dr. Damaris Grossmann

GLP-1 Success Blueprint:

Copyright © 2024 by Dr. Damaris Maria Grossmann

All rights reserved. No part of this publication may be reproduced, distributed, or transmitted in any form or by any means, including photocopying, recording, or other electronic or mechanical methods, without the prior written permission of the publisher, except in the case of brief quotations embodied in critical reviews and certain other noncommercial uses permitted by copyright law. For permission requests, write to the publisher, addressed "Attention: Permissions Coordinator," at the address below. Published By: Mindfully Integrative Dr. Damaris Maria Grossmann Rutherford, NJ Contact USA https://mindfullyintegrative.com/

damaris@mindfullyintegrative.com Published in USA

GLP-1 Success Blueprint:

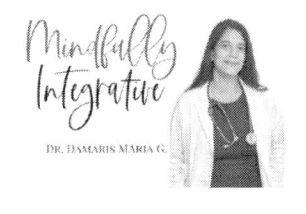

About the Author

Integrative Family Nurse Practitioner Damaris Maria Grossmann DNP FNP BSN, HNB-BC, CYN. Her Doctoral work focused on integrative health, functional medicine, and mindfulness techniques

GLP-1 Success Blueprint:

for anxiety and stress reduction for nurses, healthcare professionals, and with the use of patient care. Over 18 years in the medical field with most of those years in Nursing I am very passionate about Mindful Life Investment and Integrative Health. She has years of experience in the medical field in military, trauma, rehabilitation, college health, community health, and acute pediatric care. A US Navy Veteran served in the Global War on Terrorism in the military for almost six years and received a Navy Achievement Medal. Additionally, she studies integrative health to incorporate and facilitate her practices of Holistic modalities, in Yoga Therapy, meditation, and breathing with patient care, as a Board Certified Holistic Nurse, and as a Family Nurse Practitioner. She is a compassionate and driven nurse leader! Here to help you find a Mindful way each and every day in your optimal wellness life. She continues her studies in Functional Medicine Certification

GLP-1 Success Blueprint:

Ways to Connect: Dr. Damaris G. is an Integrative Doctor of Nurse Practice Family Nurse Practitioner Mom, Veteran, BC Family Nurse Practitioner & Holistic Integrative Health, Studies Functional & Lifestyle Medicine https://stan.store/Mindfullyintegrative

Social Media Collab/Interview/Say Hi/Email Me at

Linked In- https://www.linkedin.com/in/damarisdnp/

Website- https://mindfullyintegrative.com/

Founder- Mindful Integrative Healthcare

Office Text/Call-732-355-3469 Join our Facebook group Mindfully Integrative

GLP-1 Success Blueprint:

GLP-1 Success Blueprint:

GLP-1 Success Blueprint:

Table Of Contents

A's In Transformation   2

Introduction: Integrative Weight Management Guide for GLP-1 Users   4

Understanding the Benefits of GLP-1 Medication: 10

Conclusion: Empowering You on Your Weight Management Journey   22

GLP-1 Success Blueprint:

GLP-1 Success Blueprint:

GLP-1 Success Blueprint:

A's In Transformation

AWARENESS: This is the first step in any transformation. It's about being present in the moment and with your breathing. When you're aware of your thoughts, feelings, and actions, you can start to make changes.

ACTION: Once you're aware of what you need to change, you can start to take steps to make those changes. This could involve changing your behavior, your thoughts, or your feelings.

ALIGNMENT: This is about being centered with your heart, mind, and body. When you're aligned, you're in sync with your true self and you're able to make the best decisions for yourself.

ACCOUNTABILITY: This is about taking responsibility for your actions. When you're accountable, you're willing to own up to your mistakes and learn from them.

ACCEPTANCE: This is about being willing to accept yourself for who you are, even when you're not perfect. When you accept yourself, you're able to move forward with your life and make the changes you need to make.

GLP-1 Success Blueprint:

AUTHENTICITY: This is about being yourself, even when you're the most vulnerable. When you're authentic, you're not afraid to show your true colors and you're not afraid to be judged.

ATTENTION: This is about paying attention to detail. When you're attentive, you're able to notice things that others might miss. This can help you to make better decisions and to avoid mistakes.

ADAPTABILITY: This is about being able to adapt to different environments. When you're adaptable, you're able to roll with the punches and you're not easily thrown off course.

APPRECIATION: This is about appreciating the time, events, and circumstances in your life. When you appreciate what you have, you're more likely to be happy and content.

ABUNDANCE: This is about living your life with your means.
When you live in abundance, you're not afraid to give back and you're not afraid to receive.

GLP-1 Success Blueprint:

Introduction: Integrative Weight Management Guide for GLP-1 Users

Introduction: Integrative Weight Management Guide for GLP-1 Users

Hey there, beautiful souls! ☐ Are you ready to embark on a journey towards a healthier, happier you? As

GLP-1 Success Blueprint:

someone who has walked the path of weight management while using GLP-1 medication, I understand the challenges and triumphs that come with this process. That's why I've created this Integrative Weight Management Guide for GLP-1 Users, focusing on functional medicine and medical weight loss strategies.

Let's face it, the road to weight management can be tough, but it's essential to approach it with self-love and acceptance. ☐ Understanding the importance of embracing yourself at any weight is the first step towards sustainable change.

Through this guide, we will explore functional nutritional approaches that not only support weight loss but also enhance overall health. ☐ By incorporating these strategies into your daily routine, you'll not only see changes in your weight but also in your energy levels and overall wellbeing.

I know first hand the struggles of feeling unhealthy and obese, but there is hope. With the help of functional medicine and medical weight loss techniques, we can work towards managing our health and weight in a

GLP-1 Success Blueprint:

mindful and integrative way. It may be a long process, but it's a journey worth taking for yourself and your loved ones.

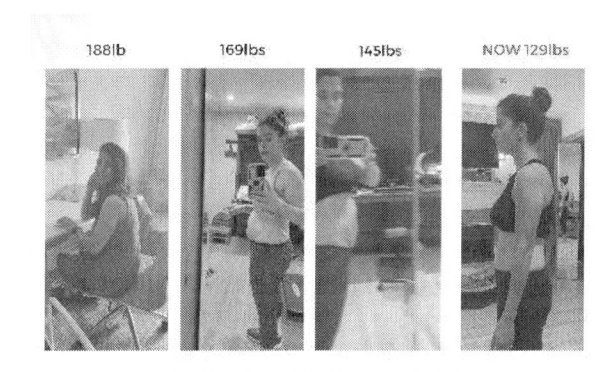

188lb   169lbs   145lbs   NOW 129lbs

WEIGHT LOSS
JOURNEY
DAMARIS GROSSMANN DNP FNP-C
HTTPS://MINDFULLYINTEGRATIVE.COM/

Together, we will dive into behavior modification techniques, nutritional recipes tailored for GLP-1 users, community support options, and so much more. Let's empower ourselves to take control of our health and achieve our weight management goals through a holistic and personalized approach.

GLP-1 Success Blueprint:

Are you ready to join me on this transformative journey? Let's do this!

#mindfullyintegrative #weightloss #functionalmedicine #selflove

Step 1: Understanding the importance of self-love and acceptance in the weight management journey

Embrace Yourself: As someone who has been on this journey, I understand the struggles and challenges that come with weight management. It's crucial to start by loving and accepting yourself just as you are. Remember, you are worthy of love and respect at any size.

One Day at a Time: Weight management is a process that takes time and patience. It's essential to approach it mindfully and integratively, focusing on small steps and progress each day. Be kind to yourself and celebrate even the smallest victories along the way.

GLP-1 Success Blueprint:

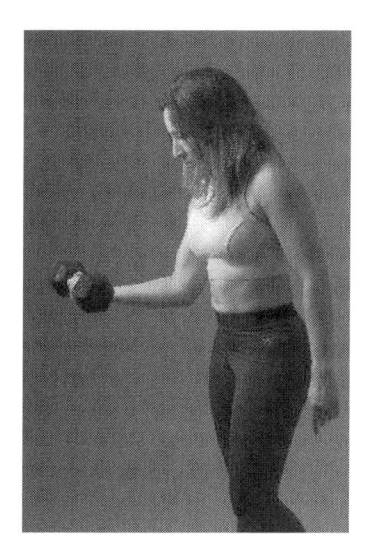

Love Yourself: Your weight does not define your worth. Whether you are at 129lbs or any other weight, it's important to prioritize self-love and selfcare. Treat yourself with compassion and understanding throughout this journey.

Hope and Healing: Recognize the importance of functional medicine and medical weight loss in addressing health issues related to obesity. It may be a long process, but there is hope for managing your weight and improving your overall well-being. Remember, you are not alone in this journey.

Mindful Approach: By incorporating mindfulness and self-acceptance into your weight management journey,

GLP-1 Success Blueprint:

you can cultivate a positive relationship with your body and food. Practice gratitude for your body's strength and resilience, and approach each day with a sense of mindfulness and self compassion.

Community Support: Surround yourself with a supportive community that understands your struggles and can provide motivation, accountability, and shared experiences. Together, we can uplift and empower each other on this journey towards better health and well-being.

Let's embark on this journey of self-love, acceptance, and holistic weight management together. Remember, you are deserving of love, respect, and a healthy body.

#mindfullyintegrative

Step 2: Exploring Functional Nutritional Approaches

Hey there, it's amazing to see you taking steps towards your health and weight management journey. As someone who has been on this path myself, I understand the importance of exploring functional nutritional approaches to support weight loss and overall health. Let's dive into some strategies that can help you along the way!

- Nutrient-Dense Foods: One of the key pillars of functional nutrition is focusing on nutrient-dense foods. Incorporating plenty of fruits, vegetables, lean proteins, and whole grains into your diet can provide essential vitamins and minerals to support your overall health and weight loss goals.

- Balanced Meals: Aim to create balanced meals that include a mix of macronutrients like carbohydrates, proteins, and healthy fats. This can help keep you satisfied, regulate blood sugar levels, and support your energy levels throughout the day.

- Healthy Fats: Don't shy away from healthy fats like avocados, nuts, and seeds. These fats are essential for brain health, hormone production, and can help keep you feeling full and satisfied.

- Hydration: Staying hydrated is crucial for overall health and weight management. Opt for water, herbal teas, and infused waters to keep your body hydrated and support your metabolism.

GLP-1 Success Blueprint:

☐ Mindful Eating: Practice mindful eating by paying attention to your hunger cues, eating slowly, and savoring each bite. This can help prevent overeating and promote a healthy relationship with food. Remember, it's all about progress, not perfection. By exploring functional nutritional approaches and making small, sustainable changes to your diet, you can support your weight loss journey and overall well-being. Keep up the great work, and remember to love yourself at every step of the way! ☐

☐

Step 3: Learning about the benefits of GLP-1 medication in weight management and how to maximize its effectiveness

Welcome to Step 3 of our Integrative Weight Management Guide for GLP-1 Users!

As someone who has struggled with weight management, I understand the importance of finding the right tools to support your journey. GLP-1 medication can be a game-changer in your weight loss efforts, but it's essential to learn about its benefits and how to make the most of its effectiveness.

GLP-1 Success Blueprint:

Understanding the Benefits of GLP-1 Medication:
Understanding the Benefits of GLP-1 Medication:

- GLP-1 medication works by regulating blood sugar levels, reducing appetite, and promoting feelings of fullness, which can lead to weight loss.
- It also has the added benefit of improving insulin sensitivity and reducing the risk of cardiovascular disease in individuals with obesity.

Maximizing the Effectiveness of GLP-1 Medication:

- Follow your healthcare provider's instructions on dosage and timing to ensure optimal results.
- Pair your medication with a balanced diet rich in whole foods, lean proteins, and fiber to support weight loss.
- Incorporate regular physical activity into your routine to enhance the effects of GLP-1 medication on metabolism and overall health.

GLP-1 Success Blueprint:

- Stay consistent with your medication schedule and lifestyle changes to see long-term benefits in weight management.

By learning about the benefits of GLP-1 medication and implementing strategies to maximize its effectiveness, you can take control of your weight management journey and achieve your goals. Remember, progress takes time, so be patient with yourself and celebrate every step forward!

Stay tuned for Step 4, where we'll dive into behavior modification techniques to help you overcome weight loss plateaus and maintain your progress. Keep up the great work! 💪

Step 4: Implementing Behavior Modification Techniques

Hey there, GLP-1 users on the weight management journey! It's time to tackle those pesky weight loss plateaus and keep making progress towards your goals. As someone who has been through it all, I'm here to share some behavior modification techniques that have

GLP-1 Success Blueprint:

helped me overcome obstacles and stay on track. Let's dive in together:

Mindful Eating: Take the time to savor each bite, listen to your body's hunger cues, and avoid distractions while eating. This can help prevent overeating and promote a healthier relationship with food.

Setting SMART Goals: Make your goals Specific, Measurable, Achievable, Relevant, and Time-bound. This way, you can track your progress and stay motivated to keep pushing forward.

Journaling: Keep a food and mood journal to identify patterns, triggers, and areas for improvement. This self-reflection can help you make more informed choices and adjust your behaviors accordingly.

Stress Management: Find healthy ways to cope with stress, such as meditation, yoga, deep breathing exercises, or engaging in hobbies you enjoy. Stress can often lead to emotional eating, so it's crucial to address this aspect of your well-being.

Accountability Partners: Connect with a friend, family member, or support group who can cheer you on, hold you accountable, and share in your successes and challenges. Having a support system can make all the difference in staying motivated.

Remember, progress may not always be linear, but with patience, consistency, and these behavior modification techniques, you can navigate through plateaus and continue moving towards a healthier, happier you. Keep up the great work, and don't forget to love yourself every step of the way! #mindfullyintegrative #weightlossjourney #behaviorchange #progressnotperfection

Step 5: Incorporating Integrative Medicine Practices for Sustainable

GLP-1 Success Blueprint:

Weight Management

Hey there, it's time to dive into the world of integrative medicine practices to enhance your weight management journey. As someone who has walked this path before, I understand the importance of incorporating holistic approaches into your daily routines for long-lasting results. Let's explore how you can integrate these practices seamlessly into your life:

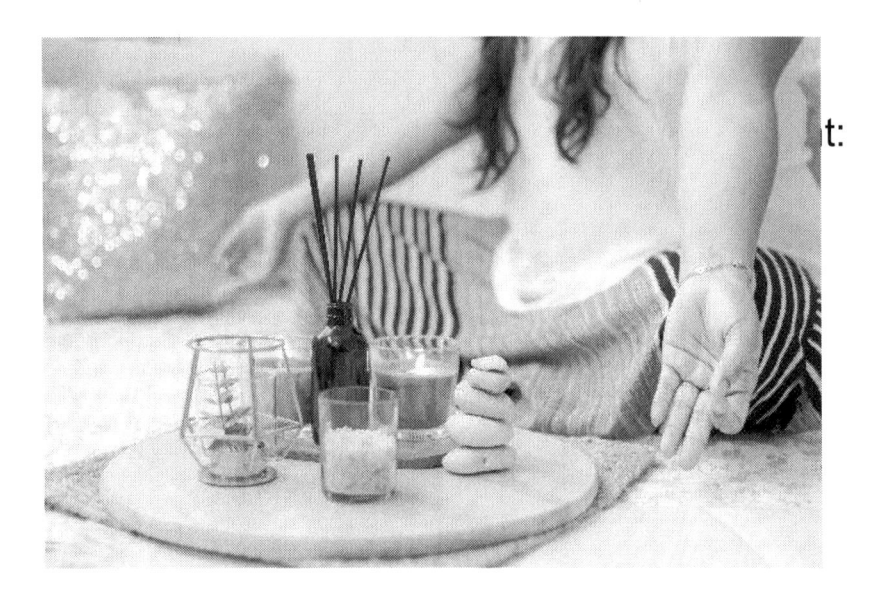

Mindful Eating: Start by practicing mindful eating techniques such as paying attention to your hunger cues, savoring each bite, and avoiding distractions while eating. This can help you develop a healthier relationship with food and prevent overeating.

GLP-1 Success Blueprint:

GLP-1 Success Blueprint:

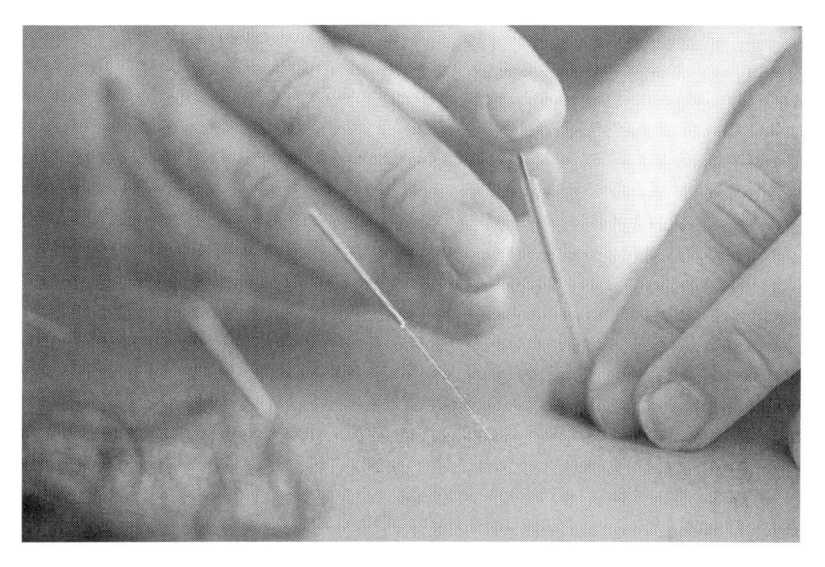

Acupuncture: Explore the benefits of acupuncture for weight management. This ancient practice can help regulate appetite, boost metabolism, and address imbalances in the body that may contribute to weight gain.

Aromatherapy: Harness the power of essential oils through aromatherapy to promote relaxation, reduce cravings, and enhance your mood. Scents like peppermint, grapefruit, and lavender can support your weight management efforts.

Chiropractic Care: Consider incorporating chiropractic adjustments into your routine to improve spinal alignment, enhance nerve function, and support overall health. This holistic approach can complement your weight management journey.

By integrating these integrative medicine practices into your daily routines, you can create a sustainable foundation for weight management that goes beyond just the numbers on the scale. Embrace these holistic approaches with an open mind and watch as they transform your health and well-being from the inside out. Stay committed, stay mindful, and remember that you are capable of achieving your weight management goals with the right tools and support. Let's embark on this journey together towards a healthier, happier you!

☐

Step 6: Trying out Nutritional Recipes Tailored for GLP-1 Users

☐ Nutrition is Key: As someone who has struggled with weight management, I understand the importance of nourishing your body with the right foods. That's why

GLP-1 Success Blueprint:

in this step, we will focus on trying out nutritional recipes specifically tailored for GLP-1 users to support healthy eating habits.

☐ Healthy Eating Habits: It's crucial to fuel your body with nutrient-dense foods that support your weight management journey. These recipes are designed to not only be delicious but also to help you stay on track with your goals.

☐ Variety is Key: One of the keys to sustainable weight management is variety in your diet. These recipes will introduce you to new flavors and ingredients that will keep your meals exciting and enjoyable.

Easy to Prepare: I know how busy life can get, so these recipes are designed to be easy to prepare, even for those with a hectic schedule. You don't have to sacrifice taste or nutrition for convenience.

☐ Balanced Nutrition: Each recipe is carefully crafted to provide a balance of macronutrients and micronutrients that are essential for your overall health and well-being. You can feel confident knowing that you are nourishing your body in the best possible way.

☐ Recipe Collection: From breakfast ideas to satisfying dinners and everything in between, this collection of recipes will inspire you to get creative in the kitchen and enjoy the process of cooking wholesome meals.

Get Cooking: So, grab your apron, gather your ingredients, and let's get cooking! These recipes are not just about eating to live but about living to eat well and thrive on your weight management journey. Let's make healthy eating a delicious and enjoyable part of your lifestyle.

Step 7: Engaging in Community Support Options for Motivation,

Accountability, and Shared Experiences

Community Support for Weight Management: As someone who has been on this journey myself, I understand the importance of having a supportive community around you. Engaging with others who are also using GLP-1 medication for weight management can provide you with motivation, accountability, and

GLP-1 Success Blueprint:

shared experiences that can truly make a difference in your progress.

Online Forums and Groups: Consider joining online forums or social media groups dedicated to GLP-1 users. These platforms can be a great source of support, where you can share your challenges, successes, and tips with like-minded individuals who understand what you're going through.

Accountability Partners: Find a buddy or accountability partner who is also on a weight management journey. Having someone to check in with regularly, share your goals with, and celebrate your victories can keep you motivated and on track.

Local Support Groups: Look for local support groups or meetups for individuals using GLP-1 medication. Meeting face-to-face with others who are on a similar path can provide a sense of community and connection that can be incredibly empowering.

Virtual Workshops and Events: Attend virtual workshops or events focused on weight management and integrative medicine. These sessions can offer valuable insights, expert advice, and a sense of camaraderie as you navigate your health journey.

Sharing Recipes and Tips: Share your favorite nutritional recipes, tips for staying on track, and strategies for overcoming challenges with your community. By exchanging ideas and experiences, you can learn from each other and stay inspired on your path to better health.

Remember, You're Not Alone: No matter where you are in your weight management journey, remember that you're not alone. By engaging in community support options, you can find the motivation, accountability, and shared experiences that will help you reach your goals and live a healthier, happier life. ☐

#CommunitySupport #WeightManagement #GLP1Users

Step 8: Embracing a mindful and holistic approach to weight loss and overall well-being

Mindful Eating: ☐

Take the time to savor each bite, chew slowly, and listen to your body's hunger cues.

GLP-1 Success Blueprint:

Be present in the moment and appreciate the nourishment you are providing your body.

Holistic Wellness: ☐

Focus on nourishing not only your body but also your mind and spirit.

Incorporate practices like meditation, yoga, or journaling to promote overall well-being.

Self-Love and Acceptance: ♥

Embrace your journey with kindness and compassion. Celebrate your progress, no matter how small, and remember to love yourself at every stage.

Community Support: ☐

Surround yourself with a supportive community that uplifts and motivates you.

Share your experiences, challenges, and successes with others on a similar path.

Functional Nutrition: ☐

Explore how food can be medicine and fuel for your body.

GLP-1 Success Blueprint:

Learn about the power of nutrient-dense foods and how they can support your weight loss goals.

Medical Weight Loss:

Trust the process and be patient with yourself.

Seek guidance from healthcare professionals who specialize in medical weight loss for personalized support.

One Day at a Time:

Remember that progress takes time, and every step forward is a victory.

Stay committed to your journey, one day at a time, and trust in the process.

Mindfully Integrative Approach:

Combine mindfulness practices with integrative medicine for a comprehensive approach to weight management.

Focus on the interconnectedness of your physical, emotional, and mental well-being.

Hope and Healing:

Believe in the possibility of transformation and healing.

Embrace the journey towards better health with hope, determination, and a holistic mindset.

GLP-1 Success Blueprint:

Step 9: Setting Realistic Goals and Tracking Progress

Setting Realistic Goals: As someone who has been on this journey myself, I understand the importance of setting realistic goals. It's essential to be kind to yourself and understand that progress takes time. Start by setting small, achievable goals that align with your overall weight management objectives. Celebrate each milestone along the way, no matter how small it may seem. Remember, every step forward is a step in the right direction.

Tracking Progress: Tracking your progress is key to staying motivated and on track towards achieving your weight management goals. Whether you prefer using a journal, a mobile app, or a wearable fitness tracker, find a method that works best for you. Keep track of your food intake, exercise routine, weight fluctuations, and any other relevant metrics. This will not only help you stay accountable but also provide valuable insights into what is working well and where adjustments may be needed.

GLP-1 Success Blueprint:

Staying Motivated: It's normal to have ups and downs on your weight management journey. Remember to be kind to yourself and stay motivated by focusing on the positive changes you are making. Surround yourself with supportive friends, family, or a community of like-minded individuals who can cheer you on and provide encouragement when needed. Celebrate your successes, no matter how small, and use them as fuel to keep pushing forward towards your goals.

On Track Towards Achieving Weight Management Objectives: By setting realistic goals, tracking your progress, and staying motivated, you are well on your way to achieving your weight management objectives. Remember that this is a journey, not a race, and every step you take towards a healthier you is a step in the right direction. Stay focused, stay positive, and believe in yourself. You've got this! #StayMotivated
#YouCanDoIt
#ProgressNotPerfection

Conclusion: Empowering You on Your Weight Management Journey

Conclusion: Empowering You on Your Weight Management Journey ~

Congratulations on taking the first step towards a healthier you! This guide was created with your well-being in mind, aiming to provide you with the tools and knowledge to take control of your health through a personalized approach to weight management. Remember, self-love and acceptance are key components in your journey towards a healthier lifestyle. Embrace who you are at any stage and know that you are worthy of feeling your best.

By exploring functional nutritional approaches and understanding the benefits of GLP-1 medication, you

GLP-1 Success Blueprint:

are equipping yourself with the necessary tools to support your weight loss goals effectively.

Behavior modification techniques will help you overcome plateaus and maintain progress, while incorporating integrative medicine practices into your daily routine will ensure sustainable weight management.

Don't forget to try out the nutritional recipes tailored for GLP-1 users to support healthy eating habits and engage in community support options for motivation and shared experiences.

Embrace a mindful and holistic approach to weight loss and overall wellbeing, setting realistic goals and tracking your progress to stay motivated on your journey.

You have the power to achieve your weight management objectives with dedication and the right strategies in place. Remember, it's a journey, not a race. Take it one day at a time and celebrate every small victory along the way.

You are capable, you are deserving, and you are on your way to a healthier, happier you. Keep going, stay

GLP-1 Success Blueprint:

focused, and never forget that your health is worth the effort. You've got this! ☐

Personalized Nutrition: Emphasizing anti-inflammatory, nutrient-dense foods to support metabolism.

Lifestyle Modifications: Tailored physical activity and stress management techniques.

Mental Health Support: Addressing emotional factors influencing weight with mindfulness and behavioral therapy.

Supplemental Support: Using natural supplements that align with GLP-1 pathways.

Comprehensive Monitoring: Regular tracking of metabolic markers and patient progress to adjust the plan as needed.

GLP-1 Success Blueprint:

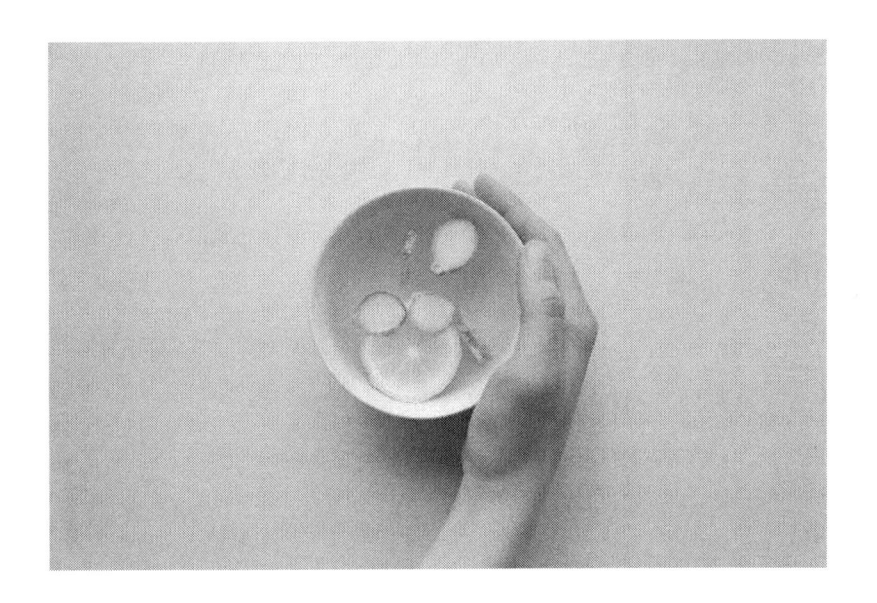

GLP-1 Success Blueprint:

GLP-1 Success Blueprint:

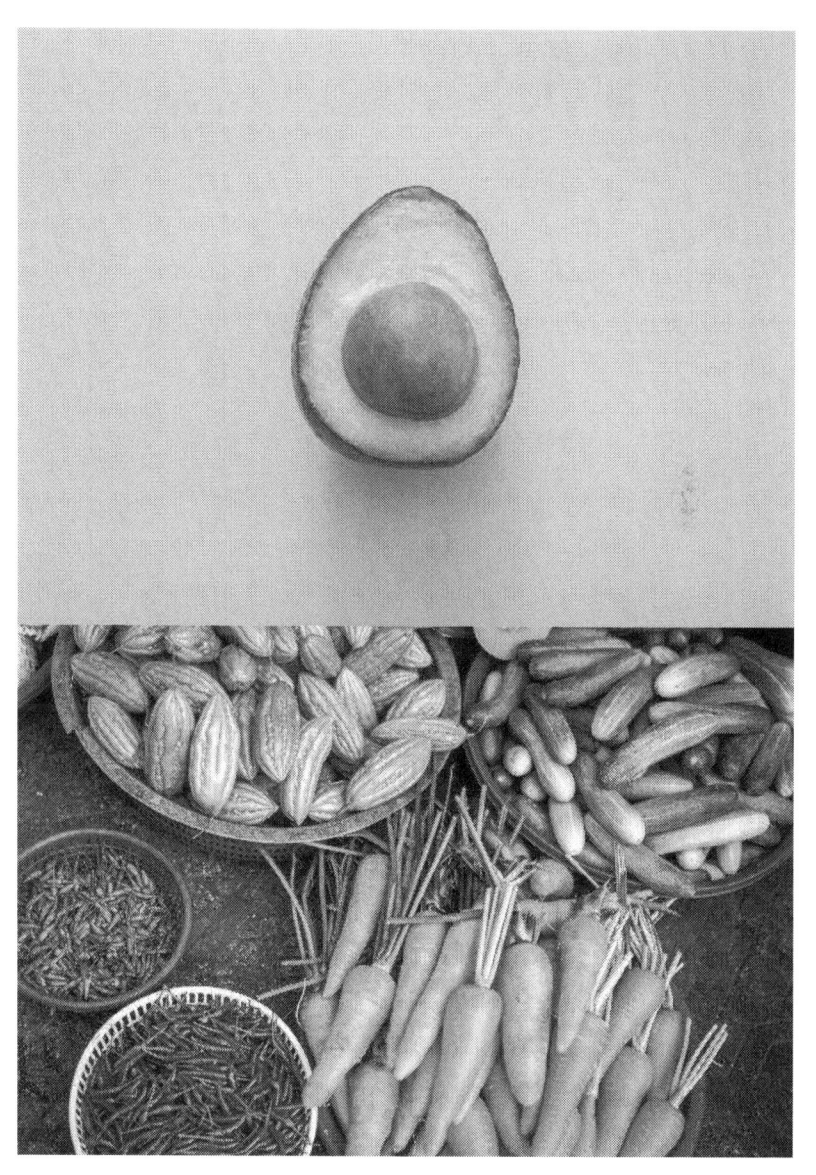

Integrative GLP-1 Recipes

Breakfast

GLP-1 Success Blueprint:

1. Green Smoothie Bowl Ingredients: 1 cup spinach, 1/2 avocado, 1/2 banana, 1/2 cup almond milk, 1 tbsp chia seeds, 1 scoop plant protein powder. Instructions: Blend all ingredients and pour into a bowl. Top with nuts and a sprinkle of hemp seeds.

2. Avocado & Veggie Omelet Ingredients: 2 eggs, 1/4 avocado, handful spinach, cherry tomatoes, sea salt, pepper. Instructions: Sauté veggies, add whisked eggs, and cook until set. Top with sliced avocado.

3. Overnight Chia Pudding Ingredients: 1/4 cup chia seeds, 1 cup coconut milk, 1 tbsp almond butter, berries for topping. Instructions: Mix chia seeds with coconut milk and refrigerate overnight. Top with berries and almond butter.

4. Greek Yogurt & Nut Bowl Ingredients: 1 cup Greek yogurt, 1 tbsp almond butter, a handful of nuts (almonds, walnuts), 1/2 tsp cinnamon. Instructions: Mix all ingredients and enjoy as a creamy, protein-rich breakfast.

5. Sweet Potato & Veggie Hash Ingredients: 1/2 sweet potato, 1/4 bell pepper, onion, 1 egg, sea salt,

pepper. Instructions: Sauté sweet potatoes, add veggies, and top with a poached egg.

Lunch

6. Quinoa & Veggie Power Bowl Ingredients: 1 cup cooked quinoa, 1/4 avocado, 1/2 cup chickpeas, spinach, cucumber, lemon juice. Instructions: Combine ingredients in a bowl and drizzle with lemon juice.

7. Spicy Tuna Collard Wrap Ingredients: 1 can tuna, 1/4 avocado, diced celery, 1 large collard leaf, sriracha. Instructions: Mix tuna, avocado, and celery, then wrap in collard leaf with sriracha drizzle.

8.Stuffed Bell Peppers with Cauliflower Rice Ingredients: 1 bell pepper, 1/2 cup cauliflower rice, ground turkey, onions, tomato sauce. Instructions: Sauté turkey and onions, mix with cauliflower rice, and fill bell pepper. Bake until tender.

9Chicken & Avocado Salad Ingredients: Grilled chicken breast, 1/2 avocado, greens, cucumber, olive

GLP-1 Success Blueprint:

oil, lemon. Instructions: Slice chicken and arrange with veggies. Drizzle with olive oil and lemon.

10. Mediterranean Chickpea Salad Ingredients: 1 cup chickpeas, cherry tomatoes, cucumber, olives, feta, olive oil, vinegar. Instructions: Toss all ingredients and enjoy as a hearty, plant-based lunch.

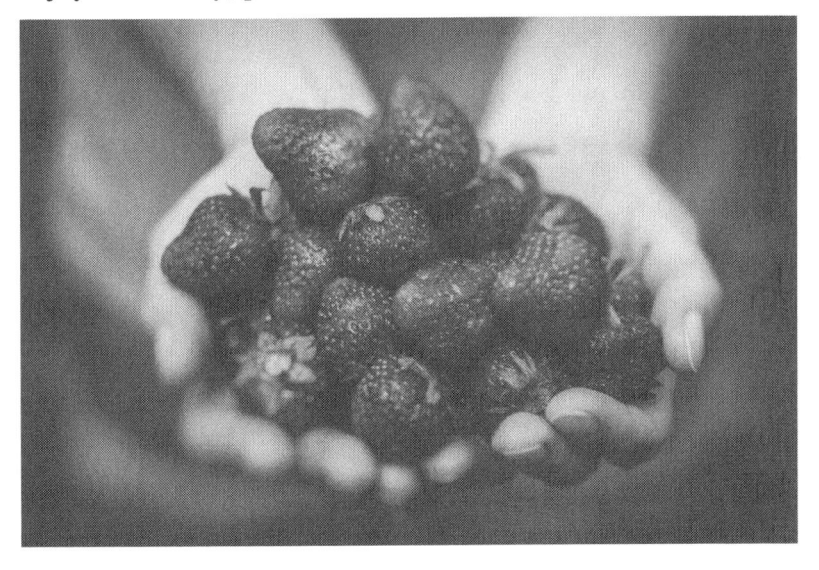

GLP-1 Success Blueprint:

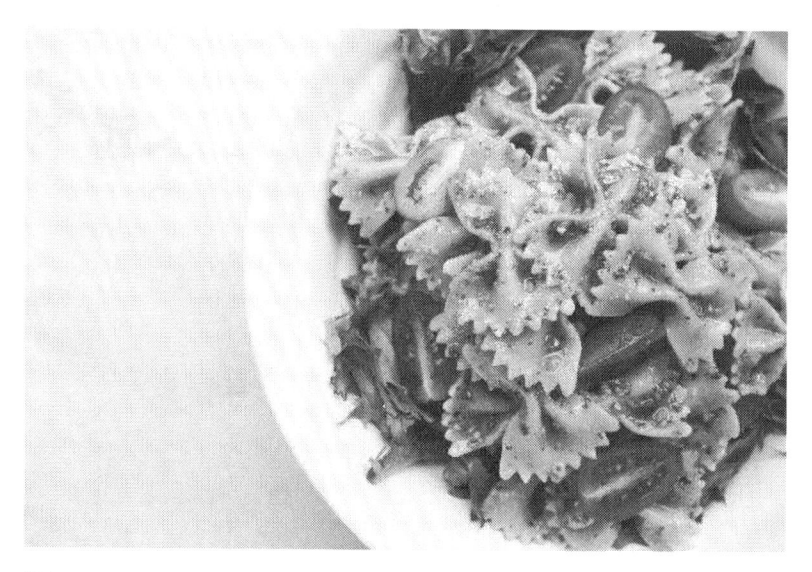

Dinner

11. Baked Salmon with Roasted Veggies
Ingredients: 1 salmon fillet, asparagus, zucchini, olive oil, lemon, garlic. Instructions: Bake salmon with veggies at 400°F for 15 minutes. Season with lemon and garlic.

12. Zucchini Noodles with Turkey Meatballs
Ingredients: Zucchini noodles, ground turkey, Italian herbs, marinara sauce. Instructions: Cook meatballs and serve over zucchini noodles with marinara.

13. Spaghetti Squash & Turkey Bolognese
Ingredients: 1 spaghetti squash, ground turkey,

marinara, basil. Instructions: Bake squash, scoop out strands, and top with turkey Bolognese.

14. Lemon Herb Chicken with Cauliflower Mash Ingredients: Chicken breast, herbs, garlic, cauliflower, olive oil. Instructions: Bake chicken with herbs and garlic. Serve with mashed cauliflower.

15. Shrimp & Veggie Stir-Fry Ingredients: Shrimp, bell peppers, broccoli, coconut aminos, ginger, garlic. Instructions: Sauté all ingredients and season with coconut aminos.

GLP-1 Success Blueprint:

Snacks

16. Veggies & Hummus Ingredients: Carrot sticks, cucumber slices, celery, 1/4 cup hummus. Instructions: Serve fresh veggies with hummus for a fiber-rich snack.

17. Almond & Berry Mix Ingredients: Handful of almonds, handful of mixed berries. Instructions: Combine for a satisfying and nutrient-dense snack.

18. Protein Energy Balls Ingredients: 1/2 cup oats, 2 tbsp almond butter, 1 tbsp honey, chia seeds, dark chocolate chips. Instructions: Mix ingredients, form balls, and refrigerate.

19. Apple Slices with Nut Butter Ingredients: 1 apple, 1 tbsp almond butter. Instructions: Slice apple and dip in almond butter for a balanced, quick snack.

20. Cucumber & Avocado Bites Ingredients: Cucumber slices, 1/4 avocado, sea salt.

GLP-1 Success Blueprint:

Instructions: Top cucumber slices with avocado and sprinkle with sea salt.

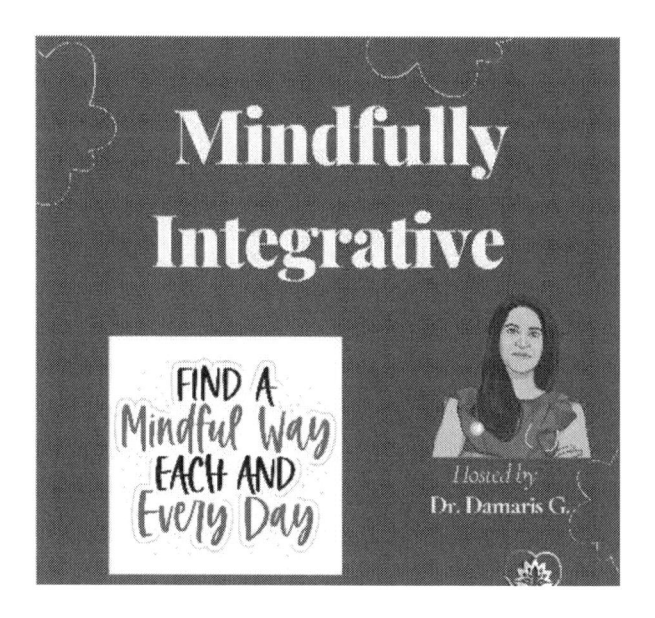

https://stan.store/Mindfullyintegrative

Enjoy https://mindfullyintegrative.com/

Fill in your Own Affirmation or Sutra

- ☐ I will try _____.
- ☐ I trust _____.
- ☐ I choose to focus on _____.
- ☐ I am ready to embrace _____.
- ☐ I am open to _____.
- ☐ I will manifest all I need _____.
- ☐ I Attract _____.
- ☐ I Am Grateful _____.

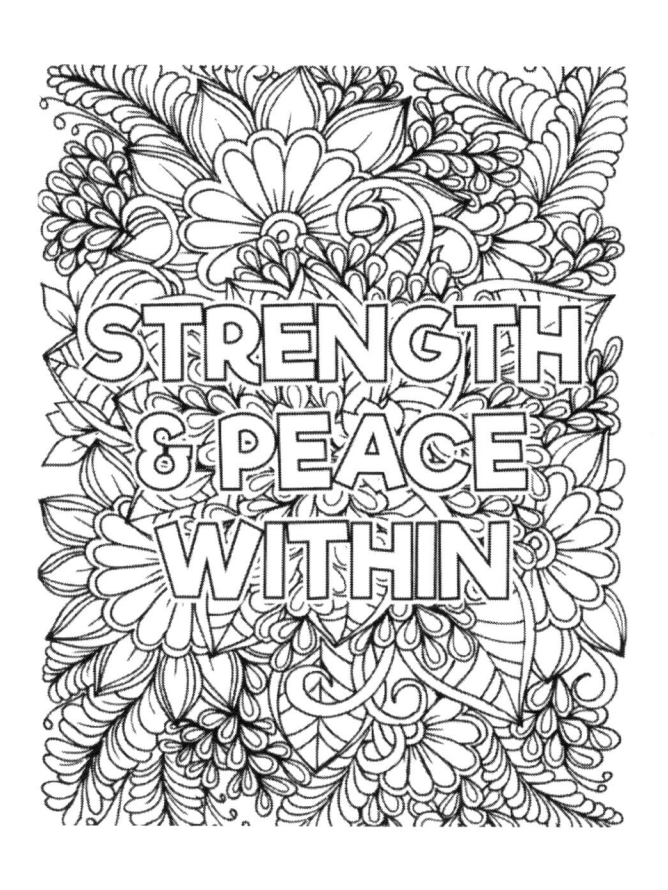

Find a Mindful Way Each and Every Day

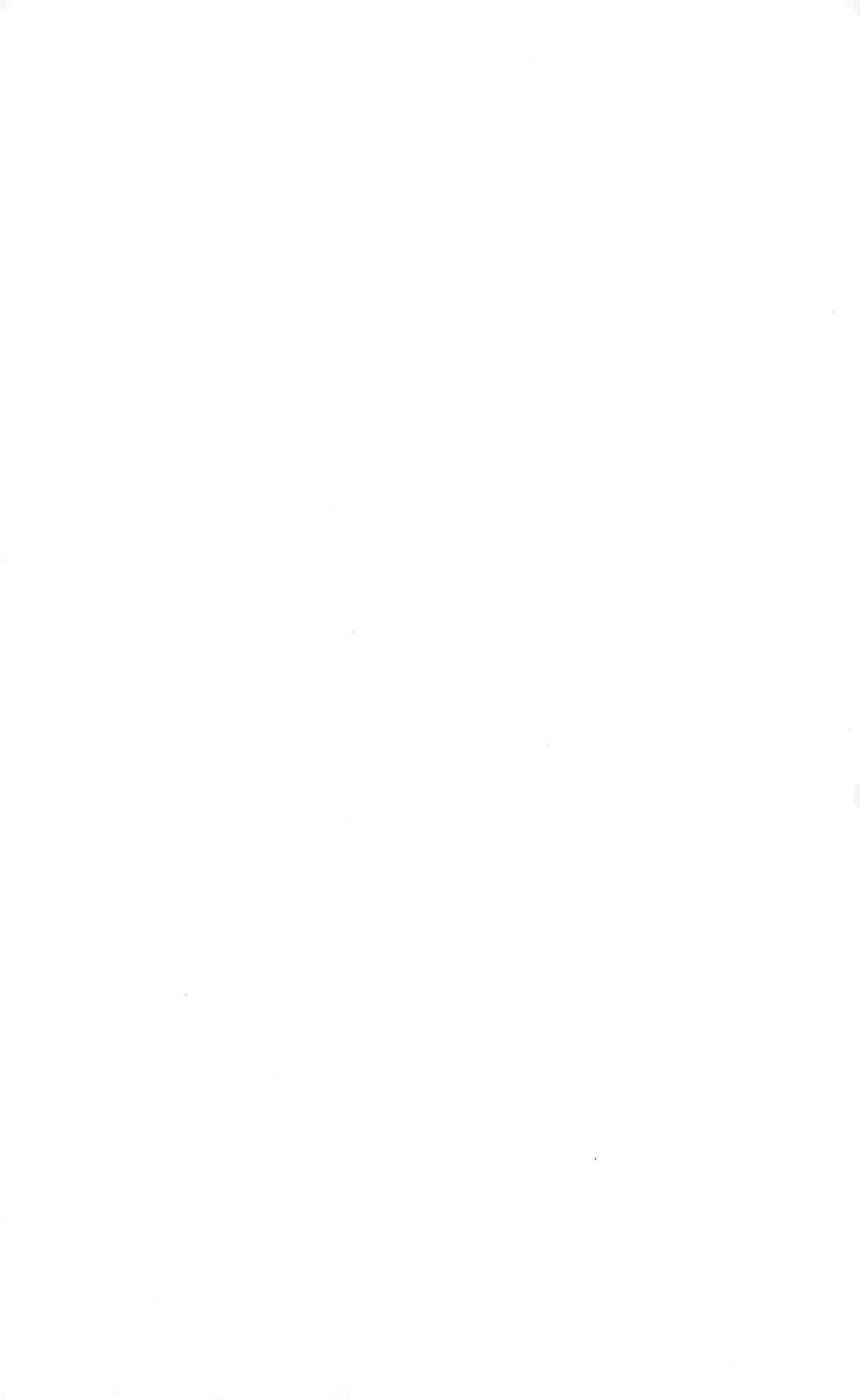

Made in the USA
Columbia, SC
02 February 2025